A Pocket Guide to Nursing Home Care

Merrilee J. Lang MSM NHA & Aleni Campos RN C-RAC

Edited by Patricia L. James MED

ISBN 13: 9781466285613
ISBN: 1466285613

Dedication

We thank our parents for their continuous support and encouragement. A special note of thanks to Mona Evans who taught me to be the best I could be, by making me believe I was almost there.

Table of Contents

Introduction

If you are reading this book it is most likely because your mom, dad, or someone else that you love has experienced an acute medical event such as a stroke, heart attack, hip fracture, or is on life's final journey requiring care and services through the support of Hospice.

While you are still trying to process the unsettling role reversal of your parents now needing your help, you will be hit with the responsibility of making key decisions that have the potential to affect the health and safety of your parent. This can be an emotionally exhausting experience for most people, but one that we hope to help you work through.

Medicare, like most health insurance programs, is designed to encourage a short stay in the hospital. So, with little warning, you will find yourself discussing with the hospital's "discharge planner" their recommendations on how to select a "skilled nursing home", or "rehabilitation center", from their preferred list of five or so facilities. With these few names and addresses you will be expected to decide on the place where your parent, spouse, or other loved one will go to receive skilled care and services while they are in their most weakened and vulnerable state.

Our intent is that the contents of this book will answer many of your questions about finding the best nursing home, as well as, provide you with information about how to navigate the complicated nursing home care systems on behalf of your mom or dad. We hope that by actively using the information provided here you will have peace of mind knowing that you have made informed decisions, using an insider's view and tips. With this advantage, you will be able to not only select the right nursing home, but to reap the maximum benefit possible out of this challenging experience!

Chapter 1

Do your homework before
going to see the nursing home

Tip: Narrow your choices down with easy research!

Once you realize that skilled nursing care is your only option, there is usually just a day or two before you must make a decision about where to send your parent. Before visiting any facilities, there are three things that you can investigate before leaving home that will help you find the right placement. You can either call the facilities and ask directly, or go online at WWW.Medicare.gov/nhcompare to check the government ratings, nursing home settings, and whether or not they will accept the payment source available to your family member.

The rating system:

The "Federal Five Star Rating" is consumer information provided by the federal government to assist people in making placement decisions. The details are complicated, but basically it is a two step system involving a formula that awards one to five stars in the areas of health inspections, staffing, and quality of care measures. Next, the stars earned in these three different categories are calculated to award each facility with one overall star rating of up to 5 stars. If a facility has earned five stars they are considered one of the best in their local market.

The nursing home setting:

Licensed skilled nursing facilities are owned and/or managed by for-profit and not-for-profit organizations. Regardless of their status, both of these offer licensed skilled nursing services in various settings. Many large retirement campuses house multiple service levels such as retirement villas, assisted living apartments, and memory care services. Other settings offer a combination of assisted living and skilled nursing under one roof, and then there are free-standing skilled nursing facilities. Excellent nursing care can be found in any of these environments, as quality of care is driven by well informed people that utilize good care systems.

The payment:

Virtually all facilities accept private payment. Most, though not all, accept Medicare and Medicaid. If the payment will be made through one of the HMO providers, it may save you money to verify the facility is within the HMO network to avoid incurring any unnecessary "out of network" charges. Keep in mind that although a facility states they accept Medicaid, all of their beds designated for Medicaid payment may be filled, and they may have a waiting list of several months. This is due to the simple fact that most Medicaid beds will be filled first with current residents who have exhausted their personal funds paying privately.

> *Tip: Take detailed notes during the tour in order to compare the facilities later!*

Chapter 2

Take a tour and see for yourself if they are good enough

As we alluded to earlier, it is wise to visit the facilities yourself to make the best decision for your loved one. Touring facilities is most telling when done unannounced, at mealtime, or during off hours. Here is a short checklist that will help you to see and understand some important features of a well managed establishment:

TAKE THE TOUR AND TAKE NOTES!

Facility #1 _____ Contact name _____ Phone # _____

Facility #2 _____ Contact name _____ Phone # _____

Facility #3 _____ Contact name _____ Phone # _____

Arrive at the facility and watch a noon or evening meal for about 10 minutes.

DINING ROOM OBSERVATIONS MARK "Y" IF THE ANSWER IS YES AND "N" IF THE ANSWER IS NO	#1	#2	#3
Look for: There is a manager or individual in charge of the dining process.			
The staff appears to be checking a card of some type prior to giving residents their food. It is critical to resident safety to ensure the proper diet and food texture is served.			
Residents are seated in groups of like ability to enhance good socialization.			
The staff engages residents in conversations, are seated when assisting residents to dine, and offer encouragement throughout the meal service.			
All residents are served water. Keep in mind that the thickness of the water may depend on the resident's ability to swallow safely.			
Residents that do not appear to be eating their food are offered substitute meal choices.			
The residents look as comfortable as possible given their physical limitations.			
The dining room is clean and the tables are pleasantly decorated with such items as linen, flowers, nice table, and glassware.			
Sound levels are appropriate and conducive to good digestion with age appropriate music playing for the resident's enjoyment.			
The food looks good to you and is garnished attractively.			
Adaptive devices, such as special plates, weighted silverware, plate guards, and scoop plates are provided to the residents to aide in their independence.			
Residents seated at the same table are served at the same time as in a restaurant setting.			

If the majority of your answers have been "yes" then proceed. If not, consider moving on to another facility. The best caregivers understand the importance of dining to a resident's mental and physical overall health and they make a point of ensuring that the dining experience goes well. Smart administrators understand that a great meal, plenty of fluids, and socialization is the first step in improving health in the senior population. Without these, seniors can experience weight loss, pressure ulcers (commonly called bed sores), and dehydration much easier than the average individual.

If the dining services meet your standards and you can see yourself enjoying a meal at the facility during future visits continue the tour.

The next step is to speak to the director of nurses, or individual in charge, to review the staffing pattern for the facility. A few important questions to ask are:

STAFFING CHECK: MARK "Y" IF THE ANSWER IS POSITIVE AND "N" IF THE ANSWER IS NEGATIVE	#1	#2	#3
What is the ratio of certified nursing assistants to residents on the day shift, evening shift, and night shift? Many states do not dictate a specific staff to resident ratio, but the bottom line is that there is enough staff to ensure the residents receive the care they deserve.			
What is the ratio of licensed nurses to residents on the day shift, evening shift, and night shift? (Ask what the state laws mandate and compare the two).			
How many open positions do they have and why? This has the potential to impact the quality of care given to the residents.			

How many contract agency staff hours have they used in the last month? Heavy use of contract labor can be indicative of poor care outcomes as there is little accountability in "here today/gone tomorrow" staff.			
What is the average tenure of the management team? This is an indicator of quality of care, proper budget-ing, and technical skill set.			
What is the average tenure of the certified aides? These are the caregivers that spend the most time with your parent/ family member.			
Do the certified aides take care of the same residents every day, or do they take care of different people every day - called "rotating"? The best care is given by people who know every detail and preference of the resident (and family) and this can only be done through the consistency of taking care of the same residents every day.			

If you are still hanging in there with the facility tour, find out the answers to these questions:

MISCELLANEOUS INFORMATION TO NOTE DURING YOUR TOUR OF THE FACILITY: MARK "Y" IF THE ANSWER IS POSITIVE AND "N" IF THE ANSWER IS NEGATIVE	#1	#2	#3
Tell the nursing staff what type of pain medication your mom/dad is taking and ask how long it will take for the medication to be available once your parent has arrived.			
Ask the facility if they offer private rooms and if there is an additional cost for the private room. A private room is a plus as a night of good sleep is important in the healing process.			
Ask what issues or problems were brought up during the last three months at the Resident Council meet-ing. Were these issues resolved? If not, move on to another facility because they do not value the resi-dent's feedback.			

Ask if the management team has a stance on limiting overtime. Exhausted people are not always patient people and wise managers decrease the potential for abuse by limiting overtime.			
Take a look at the latest government inspection results or survey. This document should be accessible to all consumers. Survey results list out the exact federal regulation, by number, that have not been met and also include the scope and severity of the non-compliance. The scope and severity indicates how widespread the problem is and how badly this non-compliance affected the residents. Simply count the number of citations that begin with "F" listed on the left side of the pages to find out the number of the statutes not in compliance and then look at the ending letter to see how badly this has affected the residents. If the total count of F tag citations is higher than 10 be cautious. If the ending letter (also known as the scope and severity of the citation) is a letter higher than "F" on the alphabet scale be very wary.			
Make sure there is no limitation on visiting hours.			
Check for locations that are conducive to comfortable family visits, especially if a private room is not available for the stay.			
Ask to see the room where your mom or dad will bathe, since most resident rooms do not have a shower. Is this centralized bathing room clean, attractive, warm, and designed for privacy?			
Make a mental note of the location of the Advocacy and Hotline posters in case you need these phone numbers later on for additional services.			
Notice if staff members wear name tags and have a professional appearance. Some companies encourage their staff to wear street clothes versus uniforms to enhance the homelike environment. In either setting the staff should look and act as professional caregivers.			
Make sure that if your loved one is terminally ill that you are welcome to stay with them as long as you want to. If the staff tells you that they will make you comfortable and feed you then you are probably in a good place.			

Ask about the smoking policy if that is a concern. Many facilities have a smoking area, but most have a no smoking policy inside the facility.			
Watch to see if staff members knock on doors or call out to residents for permission to enter their rooms.			
When walking through the facility note details of cleanliness, working light bulbs, scuff marks on the walls, and look for window and mirror brightness.			
Look at the activity calendar and compare the listings to actual events. Regulatory standards require that the two match.			
Last but not least is the "feel" of the facility. Are most of the staff friendly, smiling, engaging the residents, and making good eye contact? If not, move on because if the majority of the front line staff is not happy they probably do not have a good leadership team.			

Chapter 3

What should you bring in on the first day of admission?

> *Tip: Make sure that your mom/dad is given pain medication just prior to leaving the hospital and that the pain medication is available when they arrive at the nursing home!*

The most important thing to remember on the day of admission is the resident's prescription for pain medications. Facilities always have acetaminophen and aspirin on hand but stronger pain medications, such as narcotics, are not always available due to the stringent laws surrounding their distribution and use. If your mom/dad is currently taking a pain medication in the hospital it is imperative that you ensure this medication is given just prior to leaving the hospital and will be available to them at the facility when their next dose is due. To do this you might need to ask for a handwritten prescription for the medication from the doctor, and take it to the facility so that they can have the prescription available when your parent arrives. Often, an over the counter pain reliever will just not do the job.

> *Tip: Prepare to spend about one hour signing admission paperwork and giving copies of insurance cards and advanced directives on or before the day of the admission!*

Prior to, or on the first day of admission to the nursing home you will meet with the social worker to sign the admission contract. You may be surprised to find out that signing the admission contract involves about twenty signatures. You will also be asked for copies of your family member's Medicare card, secondary insurance cards, and advanced directives. This paperwork is required by law and is important as it documents the consent to treat, choices on issues involving care, consultant use, advanced directives, and even whether or not photographs may be taken. You will receive copies of all the documents that you sign, along with, information regarding additional charges, facility rules, instructions on how to file a grievance, and finally the rights and responsibilities of the resident.

If you have any questions or concerns now is a good time to ask about them. The individual signing the admission paperwork will be able to put you in touch with the right person to resolve any issues that you have right then and there.

If the stay will be paid through private funds the above applies, as well as, the typical requirement for initial payment upon admission. A private pay stay usually involves a 30 day advance deposit for room and board. Additional charges for nursing supplies, laundry, and beauty shop will run a month behind due to the need to verify actual use.

You may want to open up a resident fund account at this time. This is a small account set up and managed by the facility so that residents can conveniently access cash to go on activity outings.

> *Tip: Advanced Directives for healthcare decisions protect the resident's right to self-determination and may ease the potential for guilt when decisions are beyond difficult!*

The facility is required by law to ask the resident or responsible party upon admission if they have documented their health care decisions through an advanced directive. If they have not documented their wishes, the social worker will assist the cognitively able residents execute an advanced directive should they so choose to do so. If the resident is cognitively impaired, the responsible party will be asked to make healthcare decisions. Some of these decisions include whether or not a resident would want to accept cardiopulmonary resuscitation, tube feedings, hospitalization and more. It is important to note that if a resident has executed a living will, the responsible party is required to enforce the resident's wishes, as documented, not their own personal wishes.

Advanced directives may include a power of attorney, durable power of attorney, health care surrogate, living will, or guardianship papers. All of these documents are a little bit different, even if they have the same title. State laws may also differ on the capacity of each one.

In general, the *power of attorney* will only allow another individual to handle the financial aspect of the stay, whereas a *durable power of attorney* typically allows for both financial and medical decision making authority. A *health care surrogate* is the individual appointed to enforce a resident's living will, while the *health care proxy* is the individual, appointed by the facility, to make health care decisions when a resident becomes unable to make decisions for themselves. The *living will* is a document signed by the resident, outlining various health care decisions the resident has made while still capable of making medical decisions for themselves. A *Guardianship* is appointed through the court system after professional medical assessments have deemed an individual incompetent.

Individuals that fail to execute an advanced directive run the risk of having one or several relatives make decisions for them that they may not have made for themselves. Sadly, this often leads to family disputes and sometimes even litigation.

> *Tip: Making a resident's room comfortable and homelike may improve their quality of life by helping to ease the depression affiliated with the loss and comfort of personal possessions!*

On a lighter note, comfortable clothing and uplifting room décor is a must. Bring in at least seven days worth of clothing, two pair of non-skid shoes, socks, undergarments, and toiletries. Make sure that you label all items in a discreet location, with the resident's name in permanent marker, since one of the most frequent complaints from family members is lost clothing. The skilled nursing facility is required to be "homelike", so feel free to bring in personal items like blankets, throw pillows, pictures, clocks, radio, magazines, computers, and books which will enable your loved one to feel comfortable. By all means remember the adaptive devices that allowed for their independence at home. Items like big button telephones, hearing aides, glasses, magnifiers, and amplifiers greatly improve quality of life. Many facilities will allow a mini refrigerator to be brought in for snack storage. But remember there may be space restrictions if there is a roommate sharing the room. If you inquire directly, you might even find a progressive facility that allows pets to be brought in as long as they are well behaved and their vaccinations are up to date.

> *Tip: Getting to know the resident's life story will help the staff see them as the very special and unique person they are now and have always been to you!*

Don't be shy about letting the staff know how important your mom/dad is to you. Your parents may not have invented sliced bread, but they did do something incredible. They gave you life, let you keep it during your teen years, and taught you most of what you know.

So be prepared for the standard interviews when the staff will ask about their new resident's career, hobbies, interests and accomplishments. Give them the details and bring in <u>copies</u> of cherished pictures. There is nothing like a picture of your mom on her wedding day or your dad in his military uniform to really bring the message home. They were really something "in their day" weren't they! The staff do take the time to talk about these pictures and it makes them curious about reading the details of the resident's lives in their plan of care. This is exactly what you want. In a super busy environment even caring people can get sidetracked and focus on "work" instead of humanity. Your goal is to draw the staff right back into seeing your mom/dad as the unique individual they are. Success in this endeavor means better care and more attention to the important details that will translate into a higher quality of life during their stay.

If your parent has some disruptive or unusual behaviors let the staff know. If you understand what triggers the behaviors and what may ease their occurrence, make sure that information is included in the plan of care.

If your parent is used to using any type of adaptive device the staff need to know in order to make those items available if you are unable to bring them in. Devices can make a huge difference in the quality of resident's lives because they contribute significantly to a sense of independence. Losing independence can severely affect mood, outlook, and even behavior. Of course this will translate into their ability to make progress while in the facility.

It is important to let the skilled nursing team know if your parent is unable to understand english. The facility is required to provide translation for them so that they are able to make their needs known. Most facilities employ individuals from many parts of the world and chances are that one of the caregivers may speak the language that your parent is most comfortable using. If a caregiver is not available to translate there are other ways that the facility will assist your mom/dad in communicating.

Chapter 4

Meet the healthcare team!

> *Tip: The certified nursing assistant will provide the majority of the care for your loved one!*

The certified nursing assistant will be the point person taking care of your loved one's basic needs. This is the individual that will spend the most time with your mom/dad and know what is really important to them. They will do the seemingly little things that mean everything. They will know your mom/dad's likes, dislikes, pain triggers, and most intimate care needs. A good nursing assistant is worth their weight in gold. The treasured aide will take the time to get to know your mom/dad and you. They will do the little extras that make their quality of life better every single day.

Tip: Never accept the unacceptable from anyone working in the nursing home industry!

The opposite of the gifted nursing assistant is the non-caring person, punching a clock, and taking a pay-check. This type of person may say they don't have time to do their work in a caring manner, when in fact they just don't care. It is true that there are a few toads in every pond and this is true of nursing assistants as well. The certificate required to qualify for a position as a nursing assistant takes about three months or less to earn and with the pay almost twice that of minimum wage many people gravitate to the field whether they care about serving the elderly or not. If your parent ends up with one of these types of care givers, or you are just not satisfied with the nursing assistant, do not hesitate to communicate your concerns to the director of nurses, or his/her designee. Let them know that your parent needs another aide, and don't back down.

The Charge Nurse is either a licensed practical nurse or a registered nurse. All nurses are responsible for following the physician's orders to implement the resident's plan of care. Their job is to document that medications are taken and whether or not they are effective. They record the overall condition and progress of the resident as related to their individual plan of care. The nurse will be responsible for communicating with the attending physician and taking orders to ensure proper care of the resident. The registered nurse is also required to assess and document the resident's medical condition in order to inform the physician accurately and within given time-frames. Physicians depend on these reports to assist them in directing the resident's care.

The director of nursing is a member of the management team and is responsible for the overall care and services within the nursing department. This includes everything from the staff schedule to the operation of the internal quality of care systems to the evaluations and educational needs of the nursing staff.

The certified dietary manager or **diet tech** works under the direction of a registered dietician and together they are responsible to ensure a pleasant, sanitary, and even restaurant style dining experience. This sounds easier than it is, given the fact that there are many different diets, food and fluid textures and thicknesses each given to accommodate the medical conditions of the residents. A wrong diet can send a resident to the hospital or worse. In addition to the physician's order for a specific diet, the resident's preferences are taken into consideration, along with their caloric and fluid requirements. This is an involved process and one of the more likely areas where a mistake may be made. (Consider this fact: In a 100 bed facility there are a minimum of 300 chances for food related errors every single day!)

The social worker usually has a degree in social work, although some states do not require this level of education. In some states a designee may be assigned to handle the responsibilities, which usually includes limited counseling, problem solving, appointment setting, roommate assignments, room changes, advanced directive implementation, family communication, and planning a safe discharge home for the resident. If a designee is assigned the social worker role a licensed or degreed social worker may be contracted to oversee the designee's performance.

The therapist may specialize in physical, occupational, or speech therapy. Physical and occupational therapy assistants have an associates degree which qualifies them to provide treatments while working under the guidance of the therapist holding the bachelors or masters degree. The physical therapist designs the plan of care for the resident's overall physical strengthening, whereas the occupational therapist develops the plan of care for the strengthening and improvement of the finer muscle groups needed to perform tasks such as bathing, dressing, and grooming. The speech therapist holds a masters degree and is charged with developing the plan of care to enhance and strengthen the resident's ability to swallow safely, speak, and improve cognitive functions.

The maintenance director oversees the fire and disaster drills, evacuation supplies, and preventative maintenance on all equipment. This member of the management team may or may not hold a degree, but is usually certified to conduct preventative maintenance and perform repairs on, various equipment, including air conditioners, pools, generators, boilers and life safety equipment. They may also negotiate vendor contracts to perform preventative maintenance and ensure licensure on specialized equipment, such as kitchen equipment, fire alarm panels and elevators.

The activity professional is required to schedule activities according to the needs and abilities of the resident population, and document resident attendance at appropriate activities, in accordance with government guidelines. The activities department is also responsible to see that all residents receive their personal (unopened) mail timely and that all residents interested in voting are given the opportunity to vote by absentee ballot, if they are unable to go to the polls. Resident Council meetings are generally scheduled and assisted by the activity director, whose job it is to follow up with any concerns or grievances brought forth by the council. The activity director is a member of the management team and may hold a bachelors degree in recreation or occupational therapy, although many activity directors have earned a certificate through the state in order to hold the position.

The administrator is responsible for the overall operation of the business. This includes everything from the quality of care, to activities, to maintenance of the physical plant, to the financial stability of the facility. The buck stops with the administrator, as every department operates under the leadership and licensure of the administrator. In some states the law holds the administrator personally responsible for the results of the facility operation.

> *Tip: Most healthcare professionals will visit the resident right in the facility!*

Other professionals that work to provide care for the residents are known as ancillary vendors. These include the medical director, pharmacists, optometrists, podiatrists, psychologists, hospice, lab, x-ray, and possibly others. These individuals work in the facility under a contractual agreement, but unless the service is covered under Medicare Part A they will typically bill for services through their own business offices. The reason for the contract between the vendor and the facility is for the resident's convenience and protection. The goal of this in house service system is to verify that the medical professionals are qualified, licensed and insured.

> *Tip: Physicians do not visit the resident daily!*

One thing that may surprise you is that the attending physician is not required to visit the resident daily. Although some states require the physician to visit the resident within twenty four hours, this is not always the case. The physician is required to visit the resident a minimum of once per month for the first three months and then bi-monthly after that. Most care is coordinated through nursing communications with the physician via telephone, or facsimile. Physicians do visit residents more frequently if there is a particular health concern or infection.

> *Tip: Over medicating and under medicating can be detrimental to the resident and cause further decline in their physical and/or mental condition!*

Another thing that you might find interesting is that a licensed pharmacist is required to review the medication regimens monthly in order to communicate recommendations to the attending physician regarding the possibility for reducing, or eliminating medications, due to the potential for adverse medication interactions or to reduce certain types of medications that have been known to have negative, and sometimes permanent, side effects in the elderly.

All in all, you can see that there are many different professionals working to improve the life of frail seniors. As the responsible party your thoughts bring the most important perspective. All of the healthcare disciplines and professionals in the world will never know your mom/dad as well as you do. Your insight, thoughts, feelings, and opinions are invaluable in improving the quality of life for your parents. When the emotional pressure feels completely overwhelming remember that the professionals are there to help guide you through this difficult journey.

Chapter 5

Learn the jargon to understand and communicate on the same level

Acuity – is the term used to describe the medical issues affecting residents. Some examples are weight loss, pressure ulcers, dehydration, and catheter use. The law dictates that facilities are aware of what diagnosis their residents have, and to take specific actions in a timely manner to ensure the highest quality of care possible.

Adaptive device – is any type of equipment that assists the resident in achieving or maintaining their maximum independence. Common examples of adaptive devices are eyeglasses, hearing aids, big button telephones and remote controls, amplifiers, magnifying glasses, and walkers.

Advanced Directive – is a legal document that is executed by the resident in order to direct the physician and facility in the care they desire should they become unable to speak for themselves.

Administrator – in most states this individual has earned a bachelors or masters degree, has completed six months to a year internship or training program and passed state and federal exams. The license indicates the administrator understands the state and federal laws governing the industry and has reasonable judgment to manage everything from financial statements to quality of care measures.

AHCA – the agency for health care administration is the government institution that regulates the skilled nursing field. The agency oversees the industry through an initial and annual state licensure application and inspection process. AHCA conducts annual and complaint investigations in order to ensure facility compliance to federal and state statutes. Non-compliance to statutory regulations may result in citations, fines, and even a loss of licensure if the problems are not resolved within a given timeframe.

Antipsychotic – is a medication that is closely monitored in the nursing home industry. Responsible parties must be educated on the risks and benefits of using this type of medication. This medication is to be used in the lowest dose possible to achieve effectiveness, while minimizing the possibility of adverse reactions and sometimes permanent changes in functioning.

Approaches – is the industry term used to mean staff interventions used to resolve or minimize a physical or mental medical condition that a resident may be suffering from.

Assessment – is the detailed set of medical factors that a licensed caregiver will consider in order to come to a conclusion about a medical problem.

Care Plan – the plan of care developed by the facility staff is the direct result of assessments (or sets of medically related questions) answered by nursing, dietary, activity, and social service personnel regarding a resident's medical condition. These assessments target physical and mental problems that require "approaches" for improving the quality of care and life experienced by the resident.

C.D.M. – the certified dietary manager is certified in dietetics and works under a registered dietician. States vary on the requirements and capacity allowed for this position.

CEU – a certified educational unit is a formal educational hour required by various state licensing boards in order for an individual to maintain their license to work. Each profession has a certain number of hours to complete annually in order to renew their occupational license. Physicians, nurses, administrators, therapists, and certified nursing assistants all must continue their education to maintain their license, or certification.

C.N.A. – the certified nursing assistant is a position that requires anywhere from two to six months of training, depending on the state. Individuals are taught to care for residents in a manner that is safe, free from infection, and allows for as much dignity as possible. These caregivers are incredibly important to the success of the resident's quality of care and life, while in the nursing home.

D.O.N. – the director of nurses is a registered nurse with an associates or bachelors degree although a few individuals hold a masters degree or higher. The director of nurses oversees everything in the nursing department from hiring, firing, and scheduling, to staff education and implementation of resident care policies and procedures. The attitude of the nursing leader significantly influences every member of her team.

D.P.O.A. – the durable power of attorney is the legal document that in many states authorizes one individual to manage the finances and health care decisions of another.

Federal Five Star Rating - is a federal nursing home rating system that is designed to assist consumers in selecting the best nursing home in their market based on state inspections, staffing, and quality measures.

Health Care Surrogate – the individual named by the resident to act on their behalf related to health care decisions as outlined in their living will or other health care document.

In-services – staff education that is not considered a CEU. This is free education required for the licensed nurses and aides in a nursing home. In many states the facility is required to provide approximately twelve hours of education a year per staff member.

Interdisciplinary team – this team includes the nurses, aides, social services, dietary and activities personnel that recommend care approaches and implement physician orders for the resident.

Living will – a legal document that outlines the resident's care decisions related to any number of health care related areas. This may include decisions related to the use of cardiopulmonary resuscitation, artificial hydration, tube feedings, alternative diets, pain medications and even the use of oxygen if the resident is determined to be in a terminal or persistent vegetative state.

L.P.N. – these nurses have generally attended school from twelve to eighteen months and passed a state exam licensing them to practice nursing.

MAR – the medication record lists the physician's orders for medications, the required dose, and how, when, and why it is to be given. The MAR must be signed after the medication is given, provide information on effectiveness of the medication, and include an explanation if the medication is not given.

MDS - the minimum data set is a federally mandated medical assessment that seeks answers to approximately seventy physical and mental health questions that the interdisciplinary team need to understand prior to providing a plan of care.

Medical Record – this information may be stored electronically or in a binder. This record will contain billing and demographic information along with all of the documentation needed to determine every aspect of care given to a resident.

MSDS – there should be one material safety data sheet for every chemical used in the facility. These manufacturer provided information sheets instruct the staff on what to do in the event the chemical in question has posed a danger to a resident or staff member. These sheets are usually kept in one very thick binder in a central location for easy access by all personnel.

Ombudsman – a government sanctioned organization staffed with volunteers, or paid employees, whose goal is to improve the lives of the elderly through investigations of complaints and attempts to resolve grievances. They may introduce informal non-binding mediation between the facility, resident, and responsible party, depending on the state they operate in.

POA – a power of attorney is a legal document, usually pertaining to financial matters, that gives an individual authority to act on behalf of another.

Proxy – an individual who acts on behalf of a resident, within the guidelines of what the resident's wishes are believed to have been.

QA – the quality assurance process is a federal mandate and involves the facility assessing the outcomes of the care and services they provide. Unsatisfactory results are required to be action planned for improvement.

Resident – the commonly used industry term to describe individuals living in a skilled nursing facility.

Resident Roster – is a document that lists every resident in the facility and what diagnosis they have that meet specific government tracking categories. Each one of these diagnosis listed by the government also have mandated requirements for care.

Responsible Party – is the individual who has accepted the responsibility to act on the resident's behalf while the resident is living in the facility. This may be the resident himself or another individual.

Restraints – are anything that prevents a resident from moving freely at will. This may be a medication, or a physical item such as a side rail, a belted device, a chair by the bed, a bed against a wall, or even tight sheets that restrict a resident's movement. Restraints can be very dangerous and are generally discouraged. The key to determining compliance with the law requires an investigation into whether the restraint is in place to assist the resident, or is it in place simply for the staff's convenience.

RN – this nurse may have an associates or bachelors degree and must be licensed in the state in which he/she is employed.

SNF – a licensed skilled nursing facility is a business that is licensed and regulated by the federal government, through state agencies. The business operates through an annual application and fee process with initial and successive annual government inspections.

SOM – the State Operations Manual is the manual that outlines an individual state's interpretation of the federal skilled facility regulations and the survey process and paperwork required to complete the various inspections.

Surveyor – government employees that have been trained in the laws pertaining to skilled nursing facility care and services and the methodology used to determine compliance with these laws.

TAR – the treatment administration record is similar to a MAR, except that the required documentation pertains to treatments and other miscellaneous physician's orders and care reminders.

T/O – a telephone order is usually written on a three part order sheet form. The nurse transcribes the order, initials, and dates the order, and then the physician has approximately seven days to sign the form verifying they gave the order via the telephone.

Tour – is the visiting of a facility by a potential resident, responsible party, or other interested person.

Chapter 6

Use the systems to receive better care!

The admission nursing assessment . . .

Upon admission, a licensed nurse will visit your mom or dad in order to gather health information, assess them for potential medical concerns, and to note their cognitive, or mental abilities. During this time it is very important that you communicate any recent mental or physical changes to the staff. For example, if your mom/dad has lost a significant amount of weight in the last year, experienced a change in their mental capacity, or had falls at home the staff needs to know. Changes like these can place your parent at an increased risk for further decline and unnecessary suffering. If the staff knows about these risks they will be better able to address the issues right away by asking the physician for treatment orders that will decrease the risk for potential problems such as, weight loss, pressure ulcers, falls, and cognitive or mood changes.

The in-depth medical assessments and resulting care plan . . .

**Tip: Ask the Care Plan Coordinator for a copy of the plan
of care so that you will know what care is to be provided
and when it is to be provided to the resident!**

Following the charge nurse's initial in-depth assessment,
the resident will be cared for according to the physician's
orders. Unless an unusual incident or significant health
change occurs in the first few weeks the care should remain
relatively constant and documented per policy. One of
the most important routine assessments that the interdisciplinary team will complete is the minimum data set, or
the MDS assessment for short. This is an in-depth ques-
tionnaire that will allow the various disciplines on the care
team to understand the medical problems that need to be
addressed, in order to assist the resident in maintaining or
returning to their highest level of functioning. The care
plan is the resulting medical plan that is created to assist
the resident in reaching their individual health goals.

Assessments and care plans are updated at various
timeframes, depending on the resident's health and
payment status. Medicare payment requires an assessment and care plan, as appropriate, on days 5, 14, 30,
60, and 90 of the resident's stay in the facility. In most
states, a private pay or Medicaid status (financial assistance obtained through the state) requires the care
plan to be completed initially, quarterly, and annually
thereafter.

As you can see, unless a significant health change has occurred, the difference in the timing of the assessments is due to the resident's payment source. Generally, a resident using private funds or Medicaid has a more stable medical condition, whereas the resident accessing Medicare benefits has recently been hospitalized and requires skilled care. Therefore, the cost of the stay for the resident on Medicare may be up to three times as much as the cost of private pay care, therefore the government uses multiple assessments to validate and alter the level of payment to the facility on a periodic basis.

Daily meetings that affect care...

Tip: If you happen to notice a change in the resident's condition ask that the charge nurse document the change on the "24 hour Report". This communication will increase the likelihood of the change being communicated to the physician, and new orders obtained to address the change that you noticed!

In order to manage resident care outcomes, most facilities have a morning meeting to review the "24 Hour Report". This report includes any significant events, or medical changes, that have occurred within the resident population over the previous twenty-four hours. Issues of concern are reported to the physician for new orders and the responsible party is notified about the changes and consent to new treatments if there are any risks involved. Facilities with good care outcomes review results of their care systems daily to make sure that they address customer service, incidents and accidents, lab and x-ray results, new physician orders, and changes in resident ability, pain level or negative behaviors on a daily basis.

Weekly meetings that affect care...

> *Tip: Ask what new interventions are being used to address medical concerns every few weeks!*

Once a week most facilities meet to discuss the resident's most likely to, or who have actually suffered a health decline in specific areas. All facilities approach this meeting a little differently, but facilities with good inspection results review medical records and care plans to ensure that they are updated to reflect new physician orders and add care approaches to address issues such as pain, weight loss, dehydration, skin breakdown (bedsores), changes in mental status, behavioral or ability changes, falls and any type of restraints (physical or chemical). This type of close attention to the key issues affecting a resident's quality of care result in improved care, better surveys, and fewer lawsuits. You will notice a direct correlation between the quality of this private clinical meeting and the answers that you receive when asking the suggested questions in chapter seven, at the care plan meeting for your loved one.

Monthly meetings that affect care...

Well run facilities have a Resident Council meeting, Safety Committee, Medication Review and Reduction Committee and an overall Risk Management or Quality Assurance meeting once per month. These meetings are very important in determining, and correcting, any negative safety or quality of care or life trends that a facility's residents may have experienced.

Resident Council meetings are attended by the residents and usually assisted by the activity director. The residents are able to speak confidentially about any aspect of care and services. Residents may give compliments, offer suggestions, and present grievances through this meeting. The activity director is to follow up as directed by the residents. Grievances are expected to be resolved timely and the resolution is to be documented in the minutes of the next meeting.

The Safety meeting is held monthly and includes several routine topics on the agenda. Common items for review are fire drill results, staff injury investigations, safety game updates and resident accident trending. For example, all unusual events are documented on an "incident report". These confidential internal documents are analyzed in a variety of ways, but are reviewed typically by shift, type of incident/injury, by specific resident involved, and often by assigned staff member. Analyzing this data monthly gives the facility valuable information that may indicate exactly which systems, staffing levels, education, or equipment need to be updated.

The committee reviewing psychotropic medications generally involves the director of nursing, the pharmacist, and the physician. Their goal is to eliminate medications that are being given without an appropriate diagnosis and to reduce medications that have the potential for permanent adverse side effects, such as involuntary movements.

The monthly quality assurance meeting is an abbreviated version of the quarterly QA meeting, with both including routine topics on the agenda. Top notch facilities conduct in depth analysis and make systematic changes to improve the quality of the care and services in all of the departments that serve the resident's needs.

Quarterly meetings that affect care...

By law, all skilled nursing facilities must have a quarterly quality assurance meeting attended by the medical director, director of nurses, and several other facility staff members. There are no requirements regarding specific agenda items for this meeting, but facilities with good outcomes usually conduct in-depth departmental audits, track and trend infection rates, and incident and accident reports, as well as, review reports from various consultants and vendors. Negative findings are then action planned for improvement. Basically, an action plan involves staff education, new work processes for the staff, and monitoring of the results. If the results do not improve the issue should be re-action planned, as with quality improvement systems in any other business.

Chapter 7

Ask the "What / Where / When / Why" questions to get the best care!

> *Tip: Participate in the care planning process by asking the right questions to improve the care!*

There are a few basics that a person in your position needs to understand if they want to experience satisfactory care and results. The first is that the facility is required to notify the designated "responsible party" if there is a significant change in the medical condition of the resident. The second is that the risks and the benefits of any new care interventions must be explained as well. This is the perfect opportunity to influence the care results, if you know the right questions to ask.

When you are informed about a "change in medical condition," or you attend a care planning conference with the facility staff, you will want to make certain that you understand the details of the medical problems discussed, as well as, the exact treatment plan to solve or alleviate the problem at hand. Examples of significant medical changes that you should expect communication about are listed below. If you are told that your mom or dad has one of these conditions, you will want to find out if the actions listed are being taken. If an action is not in place it is a good idea to understand exactly why the option is not being considered. There may be a legitimate reason for the action not to be taken, but you should understand why something is not being done. Many items listed are considered typical care approaches because they often improve the condition of the resident:

PRESSURE SORES

SOME ACTIONS TO BE CON-SIDERED BY THE FACILITY:	NOTE QUESTIONS THAT YOU HAVE:
The resident is being cleaned, turned, and repositioned at a minimum of every two hours in order to relieve pressure on the affected area.	
The dietician has reviewed the medical record and made nutritional recommendations related to additional calories, vitamins, minerals, and/or hydration.	

If the resident is prescribed a psychoactive medication the dose is being considered for a reduction. Some medications in this category may decrease movement making skin breakdown more likely due to the potential for chemical induced lethargy.	
Labs have been ordered to determine if the resident is absorbing enough protein. Extra protein may be given as a supplement although there is no guarantee the body will always absorb it.	
If the resident is also losing weight an increase in calories, snacks, and possibly nutritional supplements is being offered at least daily.	
Verify the facility is measuring and documenting the wound(s) weekly to assess the healing progress. Ask to have the healing progress reviewed with you.	
If the wound is not healing, check to see if the treatment is being changed every 2-4 weeks. This is required by regulatory standards.	
Request that a specialized mattress be used on the bed and a cushion on the wheelchair.	
The staff move or transfer the resident with a lift or with the assistance of another staff member to avoid dragging or pulling the resident. Unprofessional transfers increase the chances of the resident's skin being sheared or damaged.	

WEIGHT LOSS ("significant weight loss" is considered 5% in a month, 7.5% in ninety days, and 10% in six months)

SOME ACTIONS TO BE CONSIDERED BY THE FACILITY:	NOTE QUESTIONS THAT YOU HAVE:
Dentures have been checked to make sure they fit properly and are comfortable so the resident is able to eat without pain or discomfort.	
The dining room environment is comfortable – not too hot, cold, loud so that the resident can relax and enjoy their meal.	
The consistency of the food is the highest texture that the resident can safely handle. Many residents will not eat as much food if it is a pureed consistency because of the appearance of the meal.	
Extra calories are given through double portions, supplements, fortified or calorie dense foods, or between meal and bedtime snacks.	
Residents are offered another meal if they don't eat the meal they first selected.	
An appetite stimulant has been considered.	
Residents with a diagnosis of depression are receiving treatment and counseling if appropriate to lift their mood.	
The staff takes the time needed to assist the resident, even if they are slow to finish their meal.	

Special adaptive devices are used by residents as needed to promote independence. (Specially designed cups, plates, weighted tableware, etc).	
Family members are encouraged to bring in specialty, cultural, or favorite foods enjoyed by the resident.	
Mealtimes are adjusted if the resident needs or desires meals at alternate times.	

PHYSICAL RESTRAINTS

SOME ACTIONS TO BE CONSIDERED BY THE FACILITY:	NOTE QUESTIONS THAT YOU HAVE:
There is a diagnosis requiring the restraint.	
The many risks of using a physical restraint, such as the increased risk of pressure sore development, loss of muscle mass, physical injuries, including death, have been explained.	
The resident is unrestrained at set intervals and range of motion, or massaging and movement, is given to the restrained limbs to avoid injury, pressure ulcers, or combative behavior.	
The least restrictive device is used, such as a velcro lap belt that the resident can release himself.	

FALLS

SOME ACTIONS TO BE CONSIDERED BY THE FACILITY:	NOTE QUESTIONS THAT YOU HAVE:
Chair and bed alarms are used as appropriate. There are many varieties to choose from and some may record a family member's voice reminding the resident to stay put until a staff member comes to assist them.	
Medications have been reviewed by the pharmacist to determine if they may cause dizziness or lightheadedness.	
A lab test has been ordered to determine if the resident has a urinary tract infection.	
The call bell response time has been checked to see if the call bell is being answered within a few minutes.	
A therapy evaluation has been ordered to try to improve the resident's balance and strength.	
The bed is in the lowest position possible to avoid severe injury in the event of a fall.	
A floor mat is in use when the resident is in bed to cushion a fall out of bed.	
Cognitively able residents are reminded to use the call light.	
Each fall is investigated related to the time, place, and reason to find a creative solution.	

The environment has been adapted to meet the needs of residents with vision problems in the following ways: a night light, contrasting paint color for bathroom wall, contrasting color of toilet seat, contrasting colors of baseboard and carpeting.	
The area where the fall occurred has been checked for lighting issues, such as too little light or a glare. This can be remedied with extra lamps and/ or by using no shine wax on the floor and light filtering draperies.	
Bedside commodes, urinals, and bedpans are available for use based on the resident's preference.	

BEHAVIORAL SYMPTOMS/ DEPRESSION/ PAIN

SOME ACTIONS TO BE CONSIDERED BY THE FACILITY:	NOTE QUESTIONS THAT YOU HAVE:
The resident has been assessed for any type of pain, including physical, emotional, and spiritual with actions taken to address the specific issue resulting in pain.	
Pain has been addressed through medication, as appropriate.	
Counseling has been ordered to address psychological pain as appropriate.	
Medications have been reviewed by the pharmacist for appropriateness and the potential for a negative interaction with another medication.	
The staff has been educated on the appropriate response to catastrophic behaviors such as screaming, yelling, biting, kicking, and scratching.	
Activity personnel are involved in providing appropriate activities prior to a behavioral outburst that may be due to boredom.	
A diagnosis is in the chart that corresponds with all medications.	
Adaptive devices are used as appropriate for the resident in the dining room to maximize independence and ease frustration.	
Adaptive devices such as glasses, dentures, hearing aides, magnifying glasses, big button phones and remotes, and reachers are available for resident use to maximize independence, ease frustration, and enable residents to enjoy life as much as possible.	

INCONTINENCE / URINARY TRACT INFECTIONS / CATHETER USE

SOME ACTIONS TO BE CONSIDERED BY THE FACILITY:	NOTE QUESTIONS THAT YOU HAVE:
The resident has been assessed to determine the feasibility for bowel and bladder retraining, if they are incontinent.	
Residents that receive tube feedings, or thickened liquids, are given additional fluids to alleviate the potential for infection and avoid dehydration.	
Labs have been obtained to determine if an infection is present and an antibiotic is ordered as appropriate.	
Catheters are only used if the resident has a diagnosis to support the use of this device.	
Pain medications are used as indicated to manage discomfort caused by unavoidable catheter use.	
The staff demonstrates competent skills in personal care cleaning techniques.	

Chapter 8

Your responses can affect the overall care and services!

> *Tip: By exercising good human relations skills, you can help achieve the best care results!*

Most people have heard the ongoing invitations on television and radio encouraging family members to seek legal counsel if they are unhappy with their loved one's condition while in the nursing home. While litigation in many states is a "heads I win, tails you lose" proposition, it is not something you will want to flaunt.

When you are frustrated with something that does not have the potential to affect your parent's physical or mental health, try to take a deep breath and consider the magnitude of the problem before you hit the roof.

For example, you might find yourself very upset because your mother's hair is not styled the way she normally wears it, or your father is not shaved by 8am like he always did at home. The mental disconnect between the vibrant picture of your parent that you carry in your heart against the reality of your parent's dependence on others for grooming may bother you more than anything else, and feel next to impossible to accept.

If details like these are of the utmost importance to you, or your parent, spend a few extra minutes with the nurses aide that is assigned to your parent. Help them to understand just how important these things are to you and your mom/dad. As hard as it is for a family member to understand, the staff work long hours in this field day after day, year after year, and occasionally have to be reminded about the dangers of becoming desensitized. Try to maintain your composure, because yelling at, or berating the staff over non-life threatening issues will only encourage a widespread disappearing act the minute you walk in the door.

On the other hand, if a staff member is unresponsive, rude, or not willing to do the "little extras", they should not be in the field of caring for seniors and you should have zero hesitation in asking for another nurse or aide.

Keep in mind that many caregivers originate from a multitude of countries and exhibit body language that may sometimes appear rude or disconcerting to a US citizen, when in fact the behavior is meant as a sign of respect for your position. For example, a lack of eye contact or a soft handshake may signify dishonesty or weakness to North Americans, when in fact these behaviors may be a sign of good manners in the caregiver's homeland.

If you have a problem with anything, remember that this is a business. Ask the right person for the assistance that you need. The aide cannot help you with your bill and the activity assistant cannot usually solve your dining problem. Just as in any other business, you will need to seek out the right professional and explain the issue. If they do not respond in the timeframe that you both agree to then contact the administrator. If the administrator is unresponsive you may want to contact the facility's corporate office, local Ombudsman, or Agency for Healthcare Administration. They will be more than happy to investigate your complaint.

The best approach to any health concern that you may have is to attend the care plan meeting. This meeting is usually held quarterly but if the resident has experienced a "significant change", the facility may invite you in to an "interim care plan meeting". If you are worried that there is a health decline or you are just concerned and want to discuss your mom/dad's health care issues, then you may request a special care plan meeting. If the facility does not agree to this request you may want to consider another facility. This is a people business and all concerns of the residents and their family members should be addressed as soon as feasible.

When you are invited to the care plan meeting, take the time and go. This is the place where any and all mental and physical care issues are discussed. Good facilities will discuss specific information about your mom/dad, from the activities, dietary, social services, and nursing perspective. They want and need your ideas added to the plan of care in order to provide the best care possible. If you think the facility team is missing the mark this is your opportunity to set them straight. If you do not attend the meeting then expect the plan of care to be less than the best. The goal is to resolve the issues, so come to the meeting with some reasonable ideas that can be discussed along with the staff's ideas for the plan of care.

If you have a family dynamics issue, it is best to keep that little gem in the family. The facility staff does not need to know that you are the only one who has taken care of mom while your greedy, selfish brother lives the big life out of state. Facilities know one thing for sure, getting involved in family dysfunction often ends with the facility on the short end of a judgment and they already pay way too much for liability insurance.

The best results occur this way. Expect professionalism and dedication to care excellence from the facility. Then do your part by being firm, fair, and pleasant. Bring in special treats, lotions, and shampoos for your mom or dad. Very often aides and other facility staff buy residents basic necessities out of their own money because they feel badly for them when family members do not provide these items. Take your mom/dad out to the mall, or a restaurant, if they can possibly go. If something is wrong tell the staff straight up what the problem is and how you think it might be resolved. Use the chain of command. Do not call the regulators every single time something minor goes wrong. They are going to ask you if you brought the issues to the administrator's attention and you will want to answer in a way that shows you are fair-minded. When the holidays come around show a little good cheer and bring in a treat for the staff and residents to share. Who wants to diet during the holidays anyway? Also, a sincere thank you never hurt anyone's motivation to continue doing a job that is difficult every single day. The last thing you should really understand is this. While some staff will not care on an emotional level about your mom/dad, many of the care team will grow to love and respect them. The smartest providers allow their aides to care for the same residents day after day. This tactic allows the aides to get to know the resident and the family member's wants, needs and desires. If they know these details, the majority of aides will go above and beyond to make sure that your parent is cared for in the way that you prefer.

Chapter 9

The government regulates
the entire industry

What is licensed by the government as a "skilled nursing facility" has been known to the general public as a rehabilitation center, nursing home, old folk's home, and other choice phrases. The history of poor care given by facilities in the past, along with the increased political power of the elderly, has given rise to the current regulatory environment.

The skilled nursing industry has evolved over the last twenty years from one of producing unsophisticated, foul smelling institutions, where the elderly went to live, suffer, and die, to an establishment rivaling nuclear power in the number of regulations and government oversight.

This shift came about as the industry was turned on its ear through a combination of the 1987 Ombudsman Reconciliation Act and the industry crushing success of trial attorneys whose windfall profits, in several states, lie in large part to a seemingly small change in the statutes, allowing litigation to proceed under a *resident rights* violation, rather than malpractice statutes. In many states, this shift from the malpractice perspective to one closer in line with a civil rights mentality nearly bankrupt the industry by facilitating huge liability awards and skyrocketing insurance rates.

Another significant step toward the nursing home of today was due to the development and implementation of the detailed "plan of care", required for each resident. The fact that the care was to be individualized meant that each resident's medical condition had to be reviewed in meticulous detail, and the issues found had to be addressed by an expert team of professionals referred to as the "interdisciplinary team" or the "IDT team". (Today, the plan of care is required to incorporate both physical and psychosocial aspects of the individual). This group of medical professionals began to be responsible for the actual medical results, or "outcomes," during the individuals stay in the nursing home. This set the stage for an expectation of improved documentation and philosophy that if the medical care was not documented then it was not done, and thus subject to citations, fines, and litigation. Medical conditions became known as "problems" and medical care became known as "approaches," or "interventions". The "care plan" became the vehicle for highlighting medical problems and describing the facility's actions to address these in order to achieve improved care results.

A more recent change, in the skilled nursing industry, is the focus on the level of accountability of the individual caregiver. In the past, licensed and certified care givers were able to come to work and go home knowing that the final responsibility for resident care would lie at the feet of their employer. This is changing quickly as the federal requirement now mandates state, and sometimes federal, background screenings prior to hiring an individual. Once an incident occurs an in depth incident and/or abuse reporting is required, which enables the government to track what happened, where, when, and how an incident occurred, and exactly who was involved in the event. In some states, the government tracks healthcare workers by social security number and license, or certificate number, in an attempt to weed out the bad apples rather than allowing poor caregivers to move from one employer to another as occurred in the past.

The same regulation and litigation that forced the industry to improve their quality of care and services is now threatening the industry as overwhelming regulations continue to expand, along with fines and litigation for non-compliance. As if regulation and litigation weren't enough, the skilled nursing industry faces challenges on other fronts as well. The high stress of a tightly regulated work environment is leading to a disappearing workforce in many parts of the country. This decline in the numbers of healthcare workers, often result in massive overtime, burn out and staggering increases on salary demands.

As expenses rise in the healthcare industry, reimbursement through Medicare has shrunk from the gluttonous "reimbursement for cost" system of years ago to a "prospective payment system" which is comparable to any other managed care entity. Making financial matters worse, many families transfer resident assets forcing facilities to accept state reimbursement, which often does not cover the cost of the care provided.

The skilled nursing industry is one of the fastest paced businesses in the United States. On average, care is now better than at any time in history. It remains to be seen how the industry will evolve to meet the pressures of decreasing reimbursement and the mind blowing costs of care and litigation.

Chapter 10

Who is going to pay this enormous bill?

Becoming elderly, sick, or just plain weak and needing someone else to care for you is something that most people refuse to think about. Needless to say, most people fail to plan for this type of living arrangement. In the past, insurance plans were expensive and provided limited coverage. These days the plans are still expensive, but the coverage has improved. The key is to find out what Medicare pays for and under what circumstances they will cover the cost of the care. Then make sure that the plan you are considering covers additional services. The best long term care insurance policies cover assisted living, skilled nursing, and even home health care.

The private cost of skilled nursing is about twice as expensive as assisted living. Today the range is somewhere between one hundred fifty to three hundred dollars a day for room and board depending on whether or not the room is private, or shared with another individual, and what part of the country the facility is located in. Additional nursing home costs will be beauty/barber, nursing supplies, incontinent supplies, safety devices, equipment rental, and offsite activity programs. The pharmacy, lab, and x-ray providers will bill separately, unless the service is covered by Medicare or another insurance plan.

Individuals with **private funds** will pay approximately sixty to one hundred thousand dollars a year for skilled nursing care and supplies in a facility. If a resident cannot afford skilled nursing care, there are government assistance programs, but access to these benefits is somewhat regulated.

Medicare Part A will pay for limited skilled nursing care under certain conditions. The individual must have been admitted to a hospital for at least three consecutive nights and then be admitted within thirty days of the hospital stay to a licensed skilled nursing facility, with an approved diagnosis that requires "skilled care". In general, the term "skilled care" means that a nurse or a therapist is required to perform the care and services, and that a lay person could not be expected to perform the tasks required. If approved, Medicare will pay 100% for the first twenty days of the stay and then the stay will be covered at approximately 80% for the next eighty days – *as long as the resident remains "skilled"*. There are no guarantees for a specific length of stay under Medicare. This is determined on a day to day or week to week basis by the interdisciplinary team. There is an appeal process if the facility states that Medicare coverage is exhausted and the responsible party does not agree. The law requires that the appeal information be given to the responsible party when the notice of Medicare non-coverage is given.

Another option for government payment to the skilled nursing facility is through the state **Medicaid** program. There are attorneys that specialize in the paperwork required for individuals to become approved for state assistance. You should be aware that money transfers to other family members so that an individual may qualify for state assistance is becoming more strictly regulated and enforced. Be very careful in selecting a nursing facility if you plan on this option. Nursing homes usually limit the number of beds reserved for state assistance because the payment can be below the cost of the care.

Government Resources

Find and compare nursing homes in your area WWW. Medicare.gov/NHCompare
Medicare 1(800) 633-4227
Area Agency on Aging 1- 800- 677-1116